POETRY
COLLECTION

MR. NOBLE

NEWMAN SPRINGS PUBLISHING
320 Broad Street
Red Bank, NJ 07701

First originally published by Newman Springs Publishing 2022

ISBN 978-1-68498-337-7 (Paperback)
ISBN 978-1-68498-338-4 (Digital)

Printed in the United States of America

This book is dedicated to two people. The first person is Elvira Anthony, my mom and the woman who gave me life and my style. I love you, Mom.

The second is Tupac Shakur. His book *The Rose That Grew from Concrete* inspired me to start writing poetries.

Preface

I'm here to enlighten and brighten the world with my energy and try to encourage those who feel as if life is too hard, to bring a different outlook to things and situations by what I write. I am doing this all while working on myself every day to become an all-around better version of myself and praying that what I've written in this book may, one day, touch at least one person to put forth a better effort in relationships, family, or just everyday life. I feel like I have fulfilled my purpose on earth if I can reach one person to do better in their life.

First Impression

One must first assimilate these words I employ so beautifully,
before they contemplate the physical appearance of me.
There's no query to if I'll make the best of our initial meeting,
'cause looks are least important, it's what's
inside that must be intriguing.
They say good things come to those who wait,
but to not make your move when impressed, can also be a mistake.
In this milieu, you'd want to identify with one's talk,
'cause he/she may look good on the out,
though inside could have a cold heart.
Me; I'm unparalleled, not the type to cause emotional protection,
just an artisan who'll permanently stamp your first impression.
So this verbal composition of being
impressed has now come to pass,
hopefully we'll blossom, not just bloom to make things last.

—Mr. Noble 8/04/2007

My Number One

Privileged I once was of calling you mine, and to think,
my heart's love hasn't wavered after all this time.
My Number One
We've had exposure to others in the distance between us,
though none can compare to the softness of her touch.
My Number One
She's everything most women can't be, mentally alone
is what I choose until face to face is our destiny.
My Number One
First in her position not one before or after, will my eyes
ever encounter another female with her stature?
My Number One
'96 of August 13th day, our eyes expressed the
energy our hearts could not yet display.
My Number One
I've now come to grasp that I'll never receive her as my wife,
still I pray for the benefit of having her pass through my life.
My Number One
Any time with her will forever be considered a wave of fun, and
no matter who, what, when, where, or why she'll always be...
My Number One!

—Mr. Noble 09/17/2006

More Than a Woman

To witness her physical one may concur a female,
as she conveys her soul, they're caught within her spell.
More Than a Woman
Recognizing communication is key to
relationships that are subdued,
not only through a lover's eye, but also a mom's too.
More Than a Woman
Her casual conversation takes me on a fruitful high,
with encouraging words, that become light
to the darkness in my mind.
More Than a Woman
She appreciates the solving of riddles, read
this to guess what it means,
a lady of stature she is, also known as the queen.
More Than a Woman
With her happy heart, resourceful mind, and helping hands,
what a great combination to blend with today's striving man.
More Than a Woman
Never one to initiate conflict, her level is much higher,
yes more than a woman, but still she burns with fire!

—Mr. Noble 04/09/2009

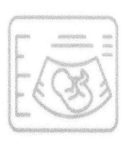
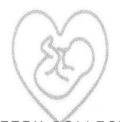
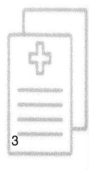

Love

Love realizes and accepts that there will be trials and tribulations,
however, with those comes a chance to express one's dedication.
It's a commitment to growth, of mind, body, and soul,
with you, I'll share this affection, so it's
worth is much more than gold.
Love is fulfillment of one another's heart,
so be the blood flow I need that keeps me out of the dark.
This is an area where fire will rise in emotions,
but don't give up, love is testing your devotion.
Like placing yourself in one another's shoes,
and finding that person with faults, still beautiful.
Love is going to your companion an admitting when wrong,
while understanding, communication will help keep the love strong.
The way she makes me feel, some may call it drugs,
'cause I'm addicted to giving and receiving true love.
Look, with love comes pain,
though as long as we see eye to eye, will forever maintain.

—Mr. Noble 07/11/2007

The Touch of a Man

This feeling is not in the physical sense of he,
but a moment of your time, and I'll
interpret to the best of my ability.
The Touch of a Man
Maturity is identified in the way one speaks,
only he brings substance to the word, by
making sure home is happy.
The Touch of a Man
Struggles alone to stand on his own two,
so, when goals are obtained they're deemed more fruitful.
The Touch of a Man
Accepting any consequence his actions may produce,
with only one to blame, he looks not for excuse.
The Touch of a Man
Sneakers, jeans, and jerseys, the look of his younger years,
now outlined in slacks, vest, and fedoras,
the appearance suggests debonair.
The Touch of a Man
When being wrong is joined with one's activity,
he has not a problem offering his apology.
The Touch of a Man
If the title threw you for a loop, it was all part of the plan,
realize characteristically you've just been schooled in
The Touch of a Man.

—Mr. Noble 04/07/2009

Elders of the World

Those who inspire, to you, I must commend,
for strengthening generations without detriment.
With you, I'll navigate the struggles of one's life,
with no thought to question counsel, I know it's sound advice.
Then, there is you who I would never seek,
because you're only the owner of age,
your actions imply, I exceed your mental page.
Your voice entails nothing of value to one's sense of vision,
however, still gaining insight through your reckless collision.
Our young are the arrows to future growth,
but to remain steady, the need is wisdom
from the elders to act as their bow.
It's not always what you preach to get them to fathom,
words are next to nil, when you lead by example.
Now to the young, please take heed to what an elder may display,
don't brush off what will turn conscious when life blows your way.
Whether old or young we're all elders who must perform,
in helping the less experienced calm their weathered storm.

—Mr. Noble 06/13/2009

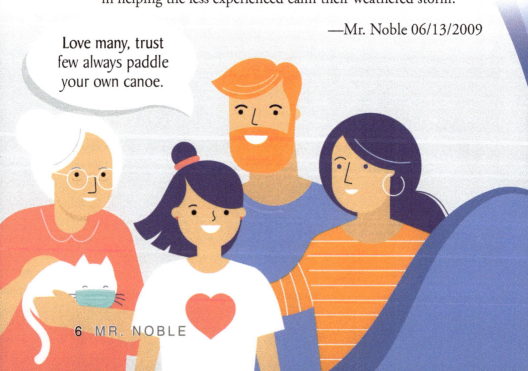

Visions

As I see the world and all its wonder,
must strive to touch skies of which I'm under.
Love of mine, soaring golden lining of the sky,
my wing is clipped so I view her flying high.
I looked up to see days turn to nights,
and just think, I used to down look stars burning bright.
To observe mountains rise gliding high with my dove,
and pluck her pink roses, its appreciation of love.
Ivory horses run wild as they beat sand,
the sky has turned dim, it's time she must land.
Her and I, colored picnics in my dreams,
sitting next to waterfalls of fresh clear water,
which turns to valley streams.
Another day has come to its end,
with me in hope of viewing ocean's waves and tides descend.
Without a torn limb, flying with my queen,
in these visions that I see,
this is truly how I wish to be.

—Mr. Noble 06/23/2009

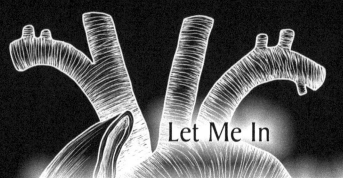

Let Me In

As I gaze into those eyes, to capture the windows of her soul,
pain is what I've grasped, in a heart that at a time
of recession it's worth more than gold.
Let Me In
Her trials and tribulations has the mind
paralleled to an "unblooming" rose,
so this new breed of soil that's at her base,
to open up to, she doesn't know.
Let Me In
Shielding her feelings, only self-inflicted they show,
holding on to the past, seemingly just stunts her growth.
Let Me In
Tried gaining her trust by being truthful indeed,
all while understanding it's earned and never given free.
Let Me In
She said, it was anger, when in truth it was more like hurt,
'cause I'd expose my existence, but of her, she wouldn't unearth.
Let Me In
So I thank you, for trying to claim the spot of my best friend,
but you must tear down that wall, for your future to begin.

—Mr. Noble 04/07/2010

You

More value than a precious timepiece,
being the worth she cannot sense, comes to me with ease.
Naive a little, and she may not want to surrender,
let life signs show you, I'm not your contender.
Hey you, why not let the fire in your blood rise?
And how can you see good in others, even through blurred eyes?
Books and learning are what intrigues her mind,
now you, help along this journey to become my queen redefined.
You have the will, however, lack a little motivation,
it's okay you, slow growth is my destination.
Puzzles to make one think is her fun,
now figure this, it is I who pushes her to be comparable to none!
In pursuit of betterment her thought of me, the world,
my burning desire for you, is to help your mind unfurl.
If this thing of ours doesn't stick like glue, then I
have not only failed myself, but also you!

—Mr. Noble 10/21/2015

Devil in Disguise

To preach of wrongdoing, while never stopping to view one's self,
pride is the advocate which prevents the asking of help.
Devil in Disguise
Deceitfulness comes natural 'cause it's executed for so long,
and when their accomplished job of betrayal
is done, it's glorified as a psalm.
Devil in Disguise
One is difficult to distinguish, with the average human eye,
'cause not only are they flesh, but also, thoughts within the mind.
Devil in Disguise
To them, their ways are true, with no room for compromise,
working through avenues of temptation, with false hope and lies.
Devil in Disguise
Their plan will cease to prosper, if we follow the path of God,
and those who don't believe consider them…
Devils in Disguise

—Mr. Noble 03/05/2009

Cut from the Same Cloth

The encounter took place when neither was looking for a friend,
brothers we are however, you wouldn't heed
by the pigmentation of our skin.
The years in which we were conceived are so distant,
you'd figure the arousal of arguments were persistent.
Altercation never has a chance to poke its nose,
due to the teachings of his forebearer, he's
looked upon as an ol' soul.
Listening and watching are the ways my lessons are comprised,
conflict doesn't exist 'cause to each other, we never lie.
In a world where loyalty is least on one's priority list,
I've found a friend who keeps it one hundred percent!

—Mr. Noble 01/15/2016

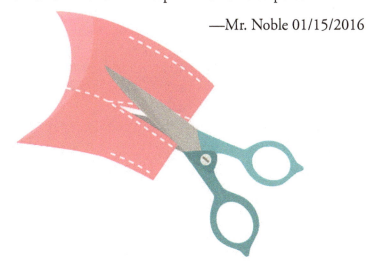

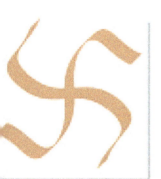

Thankful

I must start with my mom who always stayed true,
unconditionally I have her love no matter what I do.
Next let's give it up to the Lord, above,
remember his son died a terrible death to free us up.
Thankful for trials and tribulations I stand,
cause as they pass, a boy will be turned a man.
Now Malachi, is next,
being he's the motivation that fuels, this overdue process.
So I leave the negative here, and keep success in my sight,
I'm thankful for much, much more, but mostly to have life!

—Mr. Noble 08/17/2012

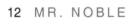

Twenty-Four/7

One whole day to celebrate the love, joy, and stress of being a mom,
however, not to lose focus, the job is 365 and never part-time.
Some women should handle motherhood a bit better,
priceless is the reproduction of life, so to all enjoy
this acknowledgment twenty-four/7.
I now hold women in a new view of admiring,
being they're the most important element to the growth of society.
At some point of this day take an hour out to
reflect on the bond of mother and child,
even in bad weather the thought should always bring forth a smile.
To me this day resides in the month of power,
rain is absent, and conceiving women are
looked upon as blooming flowers.
Those who may not have put their best
foot forward in being motherly,
understand, of your love the children are in need.
For all the mothers in the world, but especially you two,
I pray to the owner of heaven, for the protection
of my children's mom, twenty-four/7!

—Mr. Noble 05/05/2009

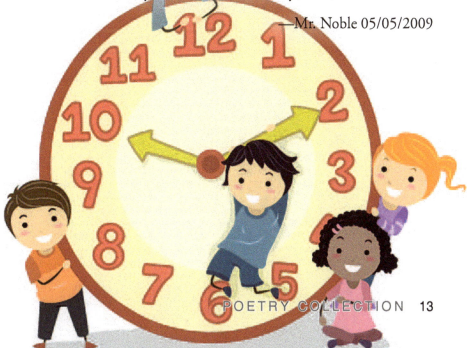

Lost

I'm lost.
Not in the sense of knowing right from wrong,
but in staying focused, to keep my foundation strong.
Comprehending the urgent process to have things my way,
though, sometimes my thoughts carry and my actions are led astray.
Growing in my second childhood, however, still considered a boy,
striving for grown man status, but lost to see its joy.
Contemplating what my uncertain mind has cost,
coming to realize it's time with he, who'll repress the lost.
Having the same eyes that stare back at me in the mirror,
to think of Malachi, everything seems much clearer.
To keep from becoming lost, means to ponder before I act.
Only to move forward, an eliminate the two steps back.
Now another slipup on my thoughts, to again become lost.
And ain't no tellin' when darkness will
come… And death will be its cost!

—Mr. Noble 10/15/2008

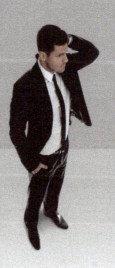

Feelings for Thee

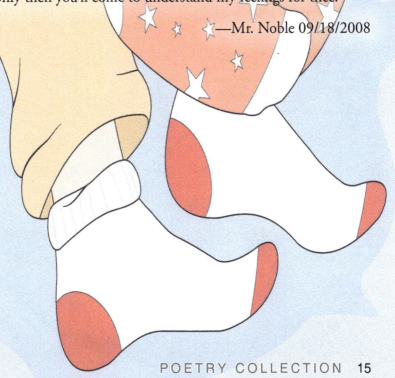

Paper is the way I express how I feel,
because verbal explanation seems to take away from my skill.
To behold how you care for others,
makes me feel the person in you, and not just as my lover.
These feelings I possess are not only physical,
intrigued with your body, though in love with the mental you.
Butterflies in one's stomach as they approach something new,
mine only seems to flutter when in contact with you.
Just the thought of gazing into your eyes,
it's like I'm caught in the dark, by a party of surprise.
Her voice entails the melody of a romantic tune,
making me feel like I've consumed a handful of mushrooms!
With her by my side the world seems less hard on me,
so please question not why the love for her is conditioned freely.
So with the issue of trust, there will be no anxiety,
only then you'll come to understand my feelings for thee!

—Mr. Noble 09/18/2008

Is There Still Time?

Has the clock stopped on what we once called beautiful?
Or does your heart still yearn for the chemistry,
a love I'll give that's true to you?
Take my time, slow it down to think, of her needs
and wants, so it's easier for our hearts to relink.
As I sit to contemplate, if there's still time, it's joined by the
little ways of how to make compromise. Thinking my selfish
actions may have clipped this lifeline, while still praying
there's a chance to learn each other, until the end of time.
This love has definitely been put to the test, but I still see growth
and development, with communication if we give it our best.
Nerdy type with glasses, so she's a little blind, yet my goal
is to hear her heart say, yes there's still time. With my heart
leading, and me killing the roaming ways of my mind,
I'll continue to self-work, until that angelic
voice never fades with time.
So if it is true, and there's still time, will you hold this in
your heart, to think what we'll be if the stars align?

—Mr. Noble 08/15/2021

This Thing of Ours

When situations prevent this thing of ours it's physical time,
the thought of me should not be held in light
with out of sight, out of mind.
Conferring attributes of a father, though a little more of a friend,
my goal is to complete you, unlike frivolous men.
Occur stern in your suggestions, even if I feel they're wrong,
your opinion accounts half as much, to
how we keep our thing strong.
Holding you in mind's eye, a smile one can detect,
while hoping to be the person behind that thought you possess.
We've indulged in one another's bodies, which is more than cool,
however, let's commence soulfully together through mental views.
This thing of ours has the potential to never grow wan,
to assist with that statement, flourish with me in spiritual bond.
Help build you up to every element I consider a queen,
of course, your reflection provides the means to which I'm seen.
Take notice when I shine, light will also smother you,
merely for the fact that in my image is how you move.
Communication is the ingredient to this
thing of ours being preserved,
accommodations with that can be matching sets of his and hers.

—Mr. Noble 05/23/2009

Pillow Talk

Sex is no forethought in our quest to confide,
so my interest lies within what stirs your mind.
As we lay, darkness enclosed,
questions are asked, discussion is made, and intimacy is exposed.
Consider this our therapeutic session,
to disclose opinions, facts, and feelings, instead of just reckon.
We're so engrossed in the world, with little time to bestow,
so the solution is pillow talk to help keep our thing in growth.
While you open up to share with me,
what's held back from the world,
I'll commence with my all to make our romance unfurl.
In this social sanctuary, arguments aren't approved,
so when we debate, it's to take in one another's point of view.
There's really no agenda to the structure of pillow talk,
though we make it stand, as a child it must walk.
To those whose relationships are skating on thin ice,
this proposal of pillow talk should work to suffice.

—Mr. Noble 08/03/2009

On My Mind

Our first encounter, a moment trapped in time,
from that day forth, what a smile has invaded my mind.
Striving for a love so strong, we'll forever be considered one,
when my thoughts relate to you, blissfulness must come.
Your sexy frame, with the way we interact, keeps you on my mind,
to view me without you, is once in a lifetime!
Visualizing you leaves me with the expression of "wow,"
and the fact of the matter is, you're on my mind now!
So important, she stimulates the brain more than money,
patient and sweet as sugar, so can I call you, honey?
Every morning I awake to question how
to get through being confined,
then a photo of you forms, my flower in sunshine.
The war within myself must come to an end,
'cause the woman on my mind is not only
a lover, but she's also my friend!

—Mr. Noble 08/24/08

Love Dedication

With the lights dimmed low,
you enter the spot with your pace extra slow.
As you move, your eyes assimilate rose petals,
from the door, to the bathroom, from the bathroom, to the bed,
don't call out, smile and take in what love has just said.
I'm now in view, and your request is an explanation,
shhh… I whisper, it's my love dedication.
Take your hands in mine, to let the feeling of
intimacy illuminate through my eyes.
I undress you, and lead you to the tub,
where arms of a bubble bath are lying in wait for a hug.
I leave, only to return with a bottle of champagne,
so after the foot massage, we'll toast to our love, despite the pain.
We're tipsy off the sparkling wine,
however, my quest is to become inebriated
from your heavenly shrine.
Assist you from the tub and dry your body off,
guide you to the bed, and commence to keeping your skin soft.
As my hands finish their teasing, we engage in locked lips,
exploring slow and sensual, so the scene is forever cherished.
Pull out all the tricks, and do more than you'd expect,
consider it Noble's play, before high-quality sex.

—Mr. Noble 04/14/2006

Father/Daddy

A Father is what I'll try my hardest to be,
not just to make babies, 'cause he's just a daddy.
A Father changes his character so his likeness can grow as a tree,
and a daddy just sees the things he wants to see.
A Father will be around through thick or thin,
Daddy just wants to see if there's an argument he can win.
Fathers spend quality time,
daddies hit you with an excuse at the drop of a dime.
Being a daddy never crossed my mind,
I'm the foundation they'll build on until the end of time.
If you're a daddy who wants to change his ways and win,
think why, get the solution, and never let it happen again!

—Mr. Noble 06/20/21

The Process

We met through a process I was always against,
not once believing, this woman may have been heaven-sent.
I put my trust in GOD, to let me know if this is real,
he answered while I read the Bible to seal the deal.
At the beginning of the process the conversation grew and grew,
now as I sit here I realize, I have those reciprocated feelings for you!
While still not knowing each other,
we put faith in the process to maybe one day become lovers.
It never occurred to me that someone so far,
could have a hold on my mind,
with that I realize to rush is not the process, we must take our time!
To learn one another to the depths of our souls,
this is the needed process for together to become one and grow old.
In this process you have to believe in words,
'cause it's distant love and she's not around
to show what you've heard.
Knowing she's been through some things,
that's why I use the process, to be attentive
and to never make her heart sting.
If the process is used and executed we shall prevail,
to saying "I do" and the permanent ringing of wedding bells!

—Mr. Noble 10/17/2021

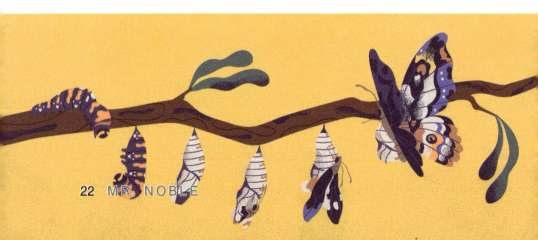

In My Mind's Eye

Seeing everything through a conscious window,
to portray life in this manner, there's less reaping of what we sow.
In my mind's eye, I try not to entertain
situations where I have no control,
only stress is caused, in a world where peaceful living is my goal.
It produces the betterment of the mind, soul, and also the physical,
to help weed out the negative affairs
through thoughts of our mental.
Removing all self-conscious actions, I was taught to be true,
realizing growth and wisdom comes about with seeing life anew.
I now laugh at foolish conduct, in my mind's eye,
it's all done in keeping the urge of conflict at its demise.
Not once degrading the behavior of those who
choose life with the substance of a rock,
just praying they'll understand, progression is
established with thinking outside the box.
These words were put together through
circumstances glimpsed by the physical eye,
broken down and analyzed by the mind, so
you'll receive this message I provide.

—Mr. Noble 03/16/2009

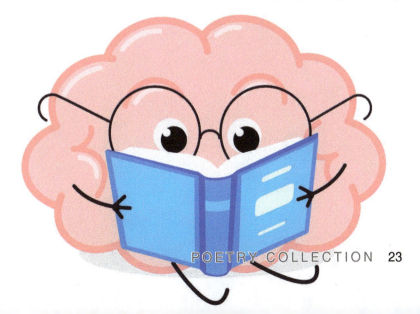

Thank You

I say this in appreciation of the things you do,
for being there for me, and just being you.
For all the great advice you've given me,
that my stubbornness blinded my eyes to see.
Thank you for being one of the best in the world,
so Mom, I owe my life to you, girl!
My heart is yours for all the bullshit we've put you through,
until I die I won't stop trying to make it up to you.
You're the only person I have with me now,
I apologize for not following that path you've laid in the ground.
As I sit and contemplate all the things I've done wrong,
the words you said, years ago comes playing through the song.
I'm blessed and I thank you for giving me birth,
but I'm crying inside for the things I've done to cause hurt.
So, you should know you are wonderful,
and for being a real mother, I thank you!

—Mr. Noble 09/23/07

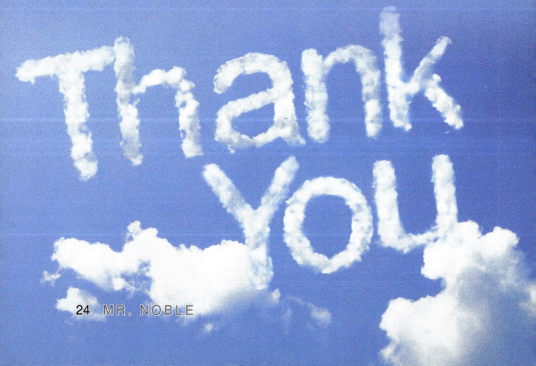

The Gift

Now the present that I speak of can't be opened physically,
everyone has their own, but they come about differently.
These gifts are with us at birth,
they may be hidden, so someone or
something must help them unearth.
See my gift is what you've read so far,
the ability to bring simple words to the
mind, like the sky does for a star.
Your gift may be something little, you might
think don't matter to someone else,
it may be the element they're looking to gather.
So listen up, you have a gift that the world needs,
now look deep within yourself pull it out and achieve.

—Mr. Noble 08/17/2012

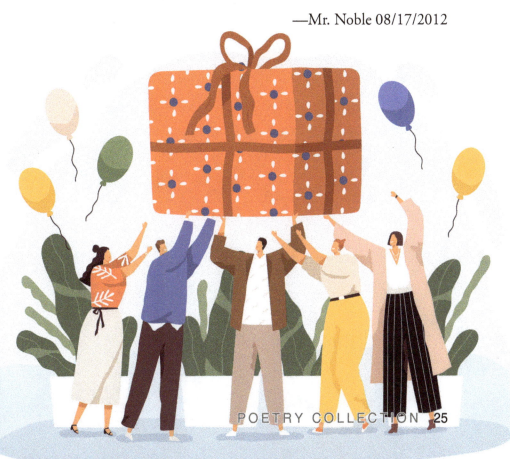

The Unknown

Where one sees no logic in the words that are produced,
even if those words are spoken in light of truth.
The unknown shakes up any promises that were made,
unwilling to view the damages it has displayed.
It's impatient and not inclined to compromise,
well, not until it can see reason through the others' eyes.

—Mr. Noble 09/16/2014

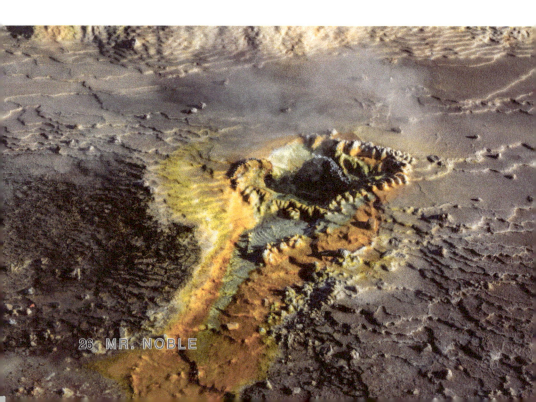

About the Author

I'm here to enlighten and brighten the world with my energy, and try to encourage those who feel as if life is to hard. To bring a different outlook to things and situations by what I write. Doing this all while working on myself, everyday to become a all around better version of myself. Praying that what I've written in this book may one day touch at least one person, to put forth a better effort in relationships, family, or just everyday life. I feel I have fulfilled my purpose on earth if I can reach one person to do better in their life.

CPSIA information can be obtained
at www.ICGtesting.com
Printed in the USA
JSHW040844050323
38435JS00007B/142